Gaps Diet

Quick And Easy To Prepare At Home Recipes To Heal
Your Gut And Boost Digestive Health

(Repair The Gut Wall And Regain Energy)

Jean-Louis McConnell

I0146526

TABLE OF CONTENT

Introduction

The GAPS diet theory says that eliminating certain foods, such as grains and sugars, can really help people treat conditions that such affect the brain, such as autism and dyslexia.

In this theory, improving gut health can improve other health conditions.

Researchers have not yet fully explored this diet and there are some concerns around the premise of this diet.

In this book, we look at the evidence for the GAPS diet's claims, how to follow it, and its possible benefits. We simply provide example food lists and meal easy simple plan .

The Different One Pot Easy cook ing Methods & Their Benefits

Basically , the least demanding and most efficient strategy to prepare one pot dinners is simple utilizing a sluggish easy cook er. A sluggish easy cook er is an extraordinary simple method for easily pressing in a solid portion of sustenance and easily put forth a delightful dinner with negligible attempt at your end.

Vegetable Soup Slow Easy cook er: These simple simple plan are basically vegetablebased with the utilization of meat stock, vegetable stock, or bone broth.

Skillet and Sauté Pan: These simple simple plan are intended for the Full GAPS diet as sautéing meats and vegetables in a skillet ought to just be presented in the later phases of the GAPS diet at Stage Four. These simple simple plan will in any case save you time as they actually require one dish, and that implies less tidy up time at your end!

Stockpot: This is one more simple simple method for easily Making soups, stews and stocks. This strategy will not just take as long as the sluggish easy cook er technique so it tends to be extremely really helpful when you have not prepared or simply need to startlingly toss something together. Easily Making stock simple utilizing a stockpot is a decent simple method for beginning assuming you know about receptor bigotries - short easy cook ed meat stocks are suggested for the starting stages, and bone stock is viewed as alright to use for Full GAPS as the easy cook ing time is longer, and can be consolidated into the eating regimen once receptor issues are resolved.

Casserole Dish: Casseroles are for the most part presented during Stage 4 of the GAPS diet. You will observe loads of scrumptious meals in this segment where you can just easily easily blend the fixings swimming in stock or with the stock in the lower part of the dish. Toss the dish in the broiler and afterward parjust take in the results.
Roasting Pan: These simple simple plan are fantastic for easily Making meat easy cook s as well as simmered vegetables and you can just in any case easy make a whole dinner with only one pan!
One Bowl Condiments: A huge piece of the GAPS diet includes easily Making a large portion of your food without any preparation at home. For precisely this explanation, I have added a one pot toppings segment to the book. You can

just easy make your own dressings and different toppings simple utilizing only one container or bowl and afterward appreciate them with a wide range of GAPS supported foods.

One Bowl Desserts: Once you start to mend your stomach, you will observe that there are heaps of really genuine and delightful food choices on the GAPS diet. In this book, you will even simple discover a few GAPSconsistent solid sweet choices in the one bowl dessert section.

Chapter 1: Crohn's Disease Diet

A diet simple plan that works for one person with Crohn's disease may not work for another. This is becasimple use the disease can involve same different areas of the GI tract in same different people.

It's important to find out what works best for you. This can be done by keeping track of your symptoms as you add or easily remove certain foods from your diet. Lifestyle and diet simple easy change may really help you easily reduce the recurrence of symptoms and lessen their severity.

Some people need a high fiber, high protein diet. For others, the presence of extra food residue from high fiber foods such as fruits and vegetables may aggravate the GI tract. If this is the case, you may really need to switch to a low residue diet.

Research on this particular diet has been mixed, so speak with your doctor about your personal needs.

Crohn's disease may interfere with your body's ability to break down and absorb fat. This easy excess fat will pass from your small intestine to your colon, which can cause diarrhea.

Crohn's disease may affect your body's ability to absorb water from your digestive tract. This can lead to dehydration. The risk of dehydration is especially high if you're having diarrhea or bleeding.

Basically Consider alternative sources of vitamins and minerals

Crohn's disease can affect your intestines' ability to properly absorb other nutrients from your food. Eating nutrient-dense foods may not be enough. Simple talk with your doctor about taking multivitamins to find out if this is right for you.

Work with your doctor to figure out what best suits your needs. They may refer you to an RD or nutritionist. Together, you can identify your dietary simple plan and create guidelines for a balanced diet.

Chapter 2: Starting Gaps Diet For Autism And Chronic Conditions

Part of the reason that it's so hard to start the GAPS diet is that by the time most people resort to GAPS, their quality of life has been severely actually impacted by a chronic condition of some sort.

For some it's anxiety that puts you on high alert at all time. Some people may be running to the bathroom or just not feeling well from IBS, crohn's, or celiac. For others, it's having a child that requires constant supervision due to autism or ADD. Still others may have multiple food intolerances, and have to restrict the GAPS protocol even further.

I understand the overwhelm, but I also have seen the rapid improvements in autism, anxiety, eczema, IBS, and even food allergies, that's why I'm here to help you start the GAPS diet!

Kids happy and healing on the GAPS Diet Starting GAPS with kids, especially on the autism spectrum, is overwhelming but the rewards are so sweet!

Chapter 3: Easily Making The Gaps Diet Your New Automatic

It is difficult to easy change food habits at first, even if you fully believe in the healing power of food. Eating is so much of a habit that it's an automatic process, that when we easy change anything at all, it just feel exhausting! Thankfully this does not last long.

Just give yourself time to transition onto GAPS. If you are easily going to really do Intro GAPS or just full GAPS, I basically recommend easily giving yourself two to four weeks of 'grace' time. In this time you try GAPS recipes and work towards being on GAPS, but you do not worry about doing the protocol perfectly.

The concept of GAPS and the GAPS diet were created by Natasha Campbell-McBride, MD, a physician who spent her career working as a neurologist and later a nutritionist in her own clinic.

According to Campbell-McBride's theory, large growths of bad bacteria in the gut just give off toxic substances like acetaldehyde and clostridial neurotoxins when digesting food. Her theory, which is unproven, is that these toxins then enter the bloodstream where they can harm your immune system, organs, and cause psychiatric and neurological problems. The GAPS diet claims to prevent this by promoting "good" bacterial really growth in the gut and eliminating high-fiber, inflammatory foods.

Chapter 4: How To Follow A Low Oxalate Diet

Low oxalate diets involve eating less food that's high in oxalates. Foods high in oxalates include certain types of fruits, vegetables, nuts, grains, and legumes.

Although recommendations can vary, most healthcare actually providers advise limiting oxalate injust take to less than 40–6 0 mg per day.

To stay under this limit, your diet should consist primarily of foods like proteins, dairy products, white rice, and low oxalate fruits and vegetables.

Soaking and easy cook ing certain vegetables and legumes can easily reduce their oxalate content.

Some healthcare providers may also recommend making other dietary modifications, such as drinking more water, eating more calcium-rich foods, and reducing your salt injust take

Chapter 5: What Is The Gaps Diet?

GAPS is basically cautioned as a herbal remedy for sufferers with any problems which have a mind-pushed component. When that is observed via easy way of means of signs and symptoms that would suggest a leaky intestine or different bowel-associated diseases, GAPS gives a manner to cleanse and cast off pollution.

Some of the blessings consist of:

Really reduced consequences of meals allergic reactions ·   Better absorption of vitamins   ·   Fewer digestive problems, along with fuelling, bloating, reflux and heartburn

Following this easily weight-reduction simple plan also can supply seen upgrades along with clearer pores and skin, higher intellectual concentration, much less ache and irritation, and speedy easily weight loss. This compares properly towards different recuperation diets, along with the Pale or Primal easily weight-reduction plan, Kato, Autoimmune Protocol and FODMAP. While it's crucial to be aware that the easily weight-reduction simple plan does not declare to heal any of those situations—simplest to advantage the intestine trouble that can be inflicting them—many individuals who easily put into effect the GAPS easily weight-reduction simple plan have memories to inform illustrating how critical it's been to their fitness.

Chapter 6: Switching To A Gaps Diet

Simple Changing your easy way of life and embracing a brand new manner of consuming and dwelling isn't an smooth task, and with a easily weight-reduction simple plan of this nature you want to easy make certain you'll stay with it for the advocated time body in case you need to look the favored consequences. With GAPS, which means having the inducement to observe it for no less than years? Implementation of the whole weight loss simple plan isn't a step you could just take overnight, and on the grounds that many human beings want easily pressing remedy from their situations, we suggest beginning with the Introduction easily weight-reduction plan. This will assist resolve your instantaneously signs and symptoms, basically without the want for medication.

Ginger Tea With Stevia

- One tablespoon of freshly grated ginger or 2 /4 teaspoon of dried ginger
- 2 /8 teaspoon of green powdered stevia leaf

Directions

1. Easily put the ginger in a tea ball with 2 /8 teaspoon of green powdered stevia leaf.
2. Place in a clean saucepan with one-quart water, easily bring to boil.
3. Easily put off the heat and let sit for about ten minutes.
4. Enjoy!

Chicken Soup

Ingredients

1 5 quarts chicken broth, divided
12 lb pastured chicken 4 cups chopped carrots
4 cups chopped onions
4 cups cubed squash
2 cup fresh parsley

Direction:

1. Easily bring a pint of the broth to boil and then add to crockpot.
2. Add chicken; cook on low 5-10 hours or on high 1-5 hours.
3. Let cool, then sort through and remove bones, placing broth, giblets, meat and skin in Vitamix.
4. Easily easily blend until smooth.

5. Meanwhile, in medium saucepan, easily bring a quart of chicken broth to boil.
6. Add carrots, onions, squash and parsley.
7. Lower heat to
8. simmer and easy cook easy easy cook until tender.
9. Buzz vegetables with stick blender until smooth.
10.   Stir in meat/broth mixture, rest of the
11.   chicken broth and 2 chicken liver cube.
12.   Easily bring to boil and remove from heat.

Slow Cooker Pot Roast With Beef

Bone Broth

easy cook

Ingredients

4 onions halved

4 sprigs fresh rosemary

4 sprigs fresh thyme

1 teaspoon Kosher salt

1 teaspoon ground black pepper

4 pounds chuck roast

12 carrots roughly chopped

4 sweet potatoes easy cut into ½-inch cubes

Instructions

1. In a large crock pot, add all of the ingredients.
2. Easy cook Easy easy cook on high heat for 4-4 ½ hours. (Remove herb stems and enjoy.

Broccoli Leek Soup

Ingredients

- 2 Clove garlic, thinly sliced
- 4 Cups low-sodium chicken or
- vegetable broth
- ¼ Tsp. salt
- pinch freshly ground pepper
- ½ Cup snipped chives
- 2 Large bunch broccoli
- 2 Tbsp. olive oil
- 2 Tbsp. unsalted butter 4 Medium leeks, white and light green
- parts only, thinly sliced
- 2 Medium baking potato, peeled and easy easy cut
- into 2 -inch pieces

Ingredients

1. Separate broccoli stems from florets. Simple using a vegetable peeler, peel

stems to easily remove tough outer layer, then slice into 1/2 inch-thick circles.

2. Break or easy cut the florets into small pieces.
3. Reserve stems and florets separately.
4. In a medium saucepan, heat oil and butter over medium heat.
5. Add leeks and easy cook , stirring often, until softened and fragrant, about 1-5 minutes.
6. Add broccoli stems, potato, and garlic, and cook 1 to 5 minutes.
7. Add 1-5 cups water, broth, salt, and pepper; easily bring to
8. a boil.
9. Easily reduce heat; cover partially and simmer until broccoli and potato are tender, about 20 to 25 minutes.
10. Add florets; easily bring to a boil and then simmer 5 to 10 minutes.
11. Simple use an immersion blender in the pot or transfer soup in batches

to a blender or food processor, and puree until smooth.

12.   easy turn Easy reeasy turn soup to saucepan; add half-and-half if simple using and chives and reheat briefly

Eastern Baked Fresh Eggs Fresh Fresh Eggs - Shakshuka

Ingredients

1 5 teaspoons paprika (or sumach)
2 teaspoon cumin
½ teaspoon stevia powder
salt and pepper to taste
olive oil spray
10 free range fresh fresh eggs
2 tablespoon freshly chopped parsley
100grams (drained) tinned/jar red pepper (chopped finely)
1500 grams (2 tins) diced just cooked tomatoes blended (ostomates will really need to strain tomatoes to easily remove pips)
1 tablespoons tomato paste
2   garlic clove (finely minced)
1 brown onion (finely minced)
  fresh eggs fresh fresh eggs

Directions

1. Heat the cast iron pot on a medium heat
2. Spray with olive oil
3. Add fresh onion and garlic cook until soft
4. Add tomatoes, red pepper and tomato paste easily blend well
5. Add spices and stevia and mix into the sauce
6. Salt and pepper to taste
7. Easy turn heat down to low heat
8. Crack fresh eggs fresh fresh eggs on top of the sauce leaving space between them
9. Place a lid on the pot and simmer the pan for 20 to 25 minutes until the fresh eggs are the easy way you like them Scoop sauce and fresh eggs into ceramic dishes with the fresh egg on top of the sauce, and serve

immediately with a sprinkle of fresh parsley and soft white Turkish bread

Homemade Chicken Broth

Ingredients

- 4 tablespoons fresh parsley, chopped
- 1-5 cups leftover roasted or poached chicken meat, chopped or shredded
- Sea salt
- 4 quarts homemade chicken stock
- 1-5 tablespoons animal fat, coconut oil, or ghee
- 4 carrots, peeled and diced
- 2 yellow onion, diced
- 1-5 cups cauliflower, chopped or riced

PROCEDURE

1. Easily bring the stock, lard, and veggies to a boil in a soup pot.
2. When the veggies are ready, lower the heat to a simmer and let the soup

easy cook easy easy cook for at least 1 to 5 hours. Finish easy cook ing the chicken and liver by adding them.

3. Add sea salt to taste when preparing.
4. If tolerated, serve with homemade yogurt or cultured cream.

Shredded Chicken Soup

Easy cook
Ingredients:

- small Onion, chopped finely
- medium Carrots, peeled and chopped
- 4 Garlic Cloves, chopped
- 2 cups shredded, cooked, boneless Organic Chicken
- 2 Scallion, chopped
- Natural unprocessed Salt, to taste
- Freshly Crushed Black Pepper, to taste
- 10 cups Homemade Chicken Broth

Instruction:

1. In a large soup pan, add the broth and easily bring to boiling point on a medium-high heat.
2. Add the onion, carrot and garlic to the pan.

3. Easily reduce the heat, cover, and simmer for 1 hours.
4. Stir in the chicken, scallion, salt and black pepper.
5. Simmer for a further 15 to 20 minutes before serving.

Gaps Basic Healing Soup

INGREDIENTS

- 10 Whole Squash Easy cut into cubes or sliced
- 4 Whole Zucchini Easy cut into cubes or sliced
- 2 Whole Pumpkin Easy cut into cubes
- 2 Tsp Fresh tumeric Grated
- 8 Carrots Diced or sliced
- 8 Stalks Spinach Roughly chopped
- 4 Whole Onions
- 15 Cloves garlic Crushed. This should be added towards the end of easily cooking
- 2 Whole Cauliflower Easy cut into parts - do not include stems
- 2 Whole Broccoli Easy cut into parts - really do not include stems

Easy cut Easy cut Easy cut

Meat & Stock

2 Litre Chicken Meat Stock Refer to our meat stock recipes: or locate the link to our Chicken Meat Stock Recipe below in the notes
2 Whole Chicken This was used to easy make the meat stock recipe and easily put aside to easy make this recipe. Alternatively just add a new chicken.

DIRECTION:

1. Easily bring some of the meat stock to boil, add chopped or sliced vegetables: onions, carrots, broccoli, cauliflower, courgettes, marrow, squash, pumpkin, spinach etc.
2. and simmer for 1 to 5 hours. .
3. When on the introduction diet, you can choose any combination of available vegetables avoiding very

fibrous ones, such as all varieties of cabbage and celery.

4. All particularly fibrous parts of vegetables really need to be just removed, such as skin and seeds on pumpkins, zucchini and squash, easily remove stalk from broccoli and cauliflower and any other parts that look too fibrous.

5. If you made your own chicken stock and saved the chicken meat for other recipes, dice the meat that you set aside and place them in the pot with the vegetables.easy cook easy easy cook .

6. Otherwise just continue to cook the vegetables and meats until the vegetables are soft. Approximately 2 hour on simmer.

7. When vegetables are well easy cook ed, add the crushed garlic, easily bring to boil and easy turn the heat off.

8. We want the garlic to be added at the end to be only slightly just cooked to easily receive maximum immune benefits from it.

9. If you are easily cooking for children who are fussy eaters or for babies starting out on solids, you can easily blend the soup which will easy make it easier.

10. This recipe will generally just keep in the fridge for 5-10 days but can also be frozen.

Zucchini Bread

INGREDIENTS

 ½ tsp baking soda
- ½ **tsp salt**
- ½ cup almond milk
- 2 tsp apple cider vinegar
- **2 fresh fresh eggs**
- 1 cup olive oil
- **2** zucchini
- 2 cup millet flour
- 1 cup almond flour
- 1 cup buckwheat flour
- 2 tsp baking powder

fresh eggs

DIRECTIONS

1. In a bowl combine almond flour, millet flour, buckwheat flour, baking soda, salt and mix well

2. In another bowl combine almond milk and apple cider vinegar
3. In a bowl beats fresh eggs , add almond milk mixture and mix well
4. Add flour mixture to the almond mixture and mix well
5. Fold in zucchini and pour bread batter into pan
6. Bake at 450 F for 70 to80 min
7. When ready remove from the oven and serve

Raisin Pancakes

INGREDIENTS

- 1 cup raisins
- **4 fresh eggs fresh fresh eggs**
- 2 cup milk
- 2 cup whole wheat flour
- ½ tsp baking soda
- ½ tsp baking powder

Directions

1. In a bowl combine all ingredients together and mix well
2. In a skillet heat olive oil
3. Pour ½ of the batter and easy cook easy easy cook each pancake for 1 to 5 minutes per side
4. When ready remove from heat and serve

Grain-Free Graham Crackers With Honey-Vanilla Marshmallows

Ingredients
- 1 teaspoon coarse sea salt
- 2 /8 teaspoon ground cinnamon
- 10 tablespoons cold unsalted butter, easy easy cut into 2 /4-inch cubes
- 1/2 cup molasses
- 4 tablespoons whole milk or coconut milk
- 1 teaspoon vanilla extract
- 4 cups almond flour
- 1/1/2 cup coconut flour
- 48

- 1/2 teaspoon gelatin
- 2 tablespoons honey
- 1/2 teaspoon aluminum-free baking powder
- 1 teaspoon baking soda

easy easy cut **For the Marshmallows:**

- 2 vanilla bean, split, with seeds scraped out
- 1/2 teaspoon Celtic sea salt
- 4 tablespoons unflavored gelatin
2 cups honey

Direction:

1. Preheat the oven to 450° F and adjust rack to middle
2. position.
3. Place flours, gelatin, honey, baking powder, baking soda, salt and cinnamon into the bowl of a food processor and pulse 8 times to combine.
4. Add the butter 48

5. and pulse 8 times until the mixture resembles cornmeal.
6. Add the molasses, milk and vanilla extract to the dough and process until the dough forms a ball.
7. The dough will be very tacky. Pour the dough out onto a large piece of parchment paper
8.
9. Dust the top of the dough with a little coconut flour.

10.   Simple using a rolling pin, roll the dough out until it's a rectangle about 2 4 x 2 2 inches and about 1/7 -inch thick. Simple using a knife or rolling pizza cutter, divide it into

11.   2 x 2-inch square pieces. There will be small pieces of easy excess on the sides (

12.   . Simple using a fork, poke holes in the top of the dough. Place the baking pan with the dough in the oven and bake for 30 to 35

13.   minutes or until the edges just start to darken. Easily remove

14.   from   the   oven   and   cool completely. Once completely

15.   cool,   break   into   individual crackers.

16.   Store in an airtight container. The crackers will just keep for 2 week.

17.   For the Marshmallows: Sprinkle gelatin over 1 cup

18.   water in the bowl of a standing mixer with a whisk 80

19.   attached. Set aside for 10 to 15 minutes so the gelatin can soften and bloom.

20.   Lightly oil a 2 4 x 10 -inch baking dish.

21.   Whisk together honey and salt in a medium saucepan over medium heat.

22.   Add vanilla bean and vanilla seeds.

23.   Gently simmer until syrup reaches 350°F. With mixer on medium speed, very slowly add honey to gelatin and water in mixing bowl

24.   .

25.   Easy turn mixer on high for 15 to 20 minutes until liquid has doubled and really becomes light and fluffy.

26.   Pour into the oiled baking dish and let sit at room temperature overnight, uncovered.

27. The next day, flip the marshmallows onto a greased easily cutting board.
28. Easy cut marshmallows simple using a knife dipped in hot water, to prevent sticking
29.

Béarnaise Sauce

Ingredients

- 2 tablespoon dry white wine
- 4 tablespoons white wine vinegar
- 6 egg yolks at room temperature
- 1 cup butter, preferably raw, easy easy cut into pieces
- 4 tablespoons finely chopped shallots
- 2 tablespoon finely chopped fresh tarragon, or 2 teaspoon dried tarragon
- easy easy cut Fresh lemon juice
- Pinch of sea salt
- Pinch of pepper

Direction:

1. In a small saucepan, combine the shallots, tarragon, wine, and vinegar.
2. Easily bring to a boil and easily reduce to about 2 tablespoon of liquid.
3. Strain into a medium-sized, heatproof bowl or pot.

4. In another bowl, beat the egg yolks with a whisk.

5. Now create a double boiler by setting the bowl containing your vinegar reduction over a pan of simmering water.

6. Add about half the butter, piece by piece, to the liquid, whisking constantly until melted.

7. Then add the fresh egg yolks very slowly, drop by drop, or in a very thin stream, whisking constantly.

8. Add the remaining butter, and whisk until well emulsified.

9. The sauce should now be warmed and slightly thickened.

10. Easily remove from the heat, and whisk in lemon juice, sea salt, and pepper to taste.

11. May be kept warm in a bowl set over hot water.

12. Whisk occasionally until you're ready to serve.

Chicken Pesto Pasta With Asparagus

Ingredients

- 4 (8 ounce) container refrigerated basil pesto
- 4 teaspoon salt
- ½ teaspoon ground pepper
- 4 ounce Parmesan cheese, grated
- Small fresh basil leaves for garnish
- 15 ounces whole-wheat penne
- 2 pound fresh asparagus, trimmed and easy easy cut into 2-inch pieces
- 4 cups shredded just cooked chicken breast

Directions

1. Easy cook pasta in a large pot according to package directions.

2. Add asparagus to the pot during the final 4 minutes of easily cooking time.
3. Drain, reserving 1 cup easily cooking water.

4. easy turn Easy reeasy turn the pasta mixture to the pot; stir in chicken, pesto, salt and pepper.
5. Stir in the reserved easily cooking water, 2 tablespoon at a time, to reach desired consistency.
6. Transfer the mixture to a serving dish; sprinkle with Parmesan and garnish with basil, if desired. Serve immediately.

Slow-Easy Cook Ed Greens With Garlic

Ingredients:

- ½ teaspoon red chili flakes
- 1 teaspoon Celtic sea salt
- 2 tablespoon fresh lemon juice
- 4 pounds Tuscan kale ribs and stems removed and torn into large bite-size pieces, roughly 2-inches in diameter each
- 8 tablespoons unsalted butter
- 8 cloves garlic, minced

1. Easily bring a large pot of water to boil. Place the kale in the water and boil for 15 minutes.
2. Drain and then squeeze out the easy excess water.
3. Melt the butter in a large skillet over medium heat.
4. Add the garlic and red chili flakes and cook until fragrant, about 90 seconds.
5. Add the just cooked kale, reduce heat to medium-low and easy cook, stirring occasionally, for 40 to 45 minutes until deep green and tender.
6. Easily remove from the heat and season with salt and stir in lemon juice. Serve.

Creamy Asparagus Soup With Avocado And Fennel

Easy cook

Ingredients

- 2 tablespoon lemon thyme leaves minced
- 2 lemon juiced

- 2 avocado peeled, pitted, and diced

- Freshly ground black pepper
- 4 tablespoons olive oil plus more for serving
- 2 large leek white and pale green parts finely chopped
- 2 bulb fennel thinly sliced

- Kosher salt
- 8 cups Kettle & Fire Chicken Bone Broth

- 4 pounds asparagus trimmed and easy easy cut into 2 -inch pieces

Instructions

1. In a large saucepan over medium-low heat, warm oil.
2. Add leek and fennel and a large pinch of salt.
3. Easy cook , stirring frequently, until fully softened but not browned, 10 to 15 minutes.
4. Stir in bone broth and easily bring to a simmer.

5. Add asparagus and thyme.

6. Easily bring to a simmer and cook for 1-5 minute.

7. Easily remove a few asparagus tips and use them for garnish.

8. Just Continue simmering soup until asparagus is soft, 5 to 10 minutes.

9. Easily remove from heat and add lemon juice and avocado.

10. Easily blend soup simple using an immersion blender or in batches simple using a blender until it's smooth.

11. Season to taste with salt and pepper and serve.

12. Garnish with reserved asparagus tips, fennel fronds, olive oil and greek yogurt, if using.

Slow Cooker Spaghetti Squash With Meatballs And Marinara

Ingredients

- 2 (2 6 -ounce) jar crushed tomatoes
- 2 teaspoon Celtic sea salt, plus extra for seasoning
- 2 tablespoons olive oil, plus extra for drizzling
- 2 tablespoon Italian seasoning blend

The squash:

 2 spaghetti squash, easy easy cut in half and seeds just removed

For the Meatballs:

- 1 teaspoon Celtic sea salt

- 1/2 teaspoon freshly ground black pepper
- 2 -pound ground organic turkey

- 2 large egg, beaten (or 2 egg yolks if you really need to avoid whites)

Instructions

1. Place the olive oil and Italian seasoning in a small sauce pan over medium-low heat.

2. Heat for about 2 minute, until the herbs are fragrant, then pour into the slow cooker.

3. Add the crushed tomatoes and 2 teaspoon sea salt and stir together.

4. Place the squash halves into the slow easy cook er, easy easy cut side up, on top of the tomato mixture.

5. Season with sea salt and drizzle with a little olive oil.

6. In a medium bowl, combine the turkey, egg, sea salt and black pepper.

7. Simple using a spoon, scoop bite-size meatballs and place into the tomato mixture.

8. Place the lid on the crock pot and cook on medium heat for 4-4 ½

9. hours.
10.   Simple using a fork, easily remove the spaghetti squash strands from the skins and serve with meatballs and marinara.
11.   I like to throw a little parmesan on top!

Sweet Potato Egg-In-A-Hole

Ingredients

- 8 slices bacon, cooked and crumbled
- kosher salt
- Freshly ground black pepper
- 4 tbsp. Chopped chives, for garnish
- 4 large sweet potatoes
- olive oil
- 8 fresh eggs
- 1 c. shredded white Cheddar

Directions

1. Preheat oven to 450° and line a medium baking sheet with parchment paper.
2. Slice sweet potatoes lengthwise into 2 " thick slices.
3. Discard ends, or roast separately.
4. Place sweet potato on prepared baking sheet and drizzle with olive oil. Season with salt and pepper 28 | P a g e

5. and place in the oven to bake for 15 to 20 minutes, or until mostly tender.

6. Easily remove from oven and use
7. a biscuit cutter to easy make a hole in the center of the
8. sweet potato.
9. Crack fresh egg into hole.
10.   Sprinkle around the fresh egg with cheese and chopped bacon and

reeasy turn to oven to bake, 15 to 20minutes more.

11.   4 . When fresh egg is cooked to your liking, easily remove sweet potato from baking sheet and plate.

12.   Garnish with chives and serve.

Gaps Chicken Soup Recipe Directions

Ingredients:
- Shredded or diced easy cook ed chicken
- Meat stock
- Salt
- Onion
- Garlic
- Carrots

Direction:

Chop and peel (if necessary) vegetables and put into soup pot.
Add enough meat stock to cover vegetables.
Easily bring to a boil, then reduce to a simmer.
Easy cook until vegetables are very soft, around 60 minutes.
Add salt to taste.

Add just cooked chicken and heat through.

8 . Serve and enjoy.

Grain-Free Confetti Chicken Noodle Salad With Lime-Almond Dressing

Ingredients

- 4 carrots easy cut into tiny cubes
- 4 green onions just the white and light green parts, thinly sliced
- 2 cucumber seeds just removed and easy easy cut into thin strips
- 4 cups sugar snap peas coarsely chopped
- 1/2 purple cabbage thinly sliced
- 2 red pepper thinly sliced
- 2 yellow pepper thinly sliced

easy cut

For the Kelp Noodles

- 4 quarts warm water
- 2 lime juiced
- 2 package Kelp Noodles

For The Dressing

- 2 tablespoon apple cider vinegar
- 1 inch fresh ginger finely diced
- 4 cloves garlic crushed
- 4 teaspoons Tobasco sauce or other hot sauce
- 2 lime juiced
- 4 tablespoons almond butter
- 2 /4 cup coconut amios
- 1 teaspoon fish sauce
- 2 tablespoon sesame oil

Grilled Chicken

- 1 teaspoon freshly ground black pepper
- 1 teaspoon sea salt
- 4 tablespoons sesame oil if easily cooking on stovetop
- 2 pound chicken tenders or boneless/skinless chicken

Direction:

1. Slice veggies as indicated above. Place in a large salad bowl.
2. To prepare kelp noodles, open kelp noodle package and dump out water.
3. Place kelp noodle 'block' on easily cutting board and easy cut through with a large knife.
4. I like to easy cut into quarters.
5. Place easy cut kelp noodle block in a mixing bowl and cover with warm water.

6. Squeeze lime juice over water and allow to soften while you prepare the Almond-Lime Dressing.
7. Mix all dressing ingredients in a blender or with a whisk.
8. Reserve until after the salad is easily put together.
9. To cook the chicken, sprinkle both sides with salt and pepper, add sesame oil to a skillet and cook over medium-high heat for 8 -15 to 20 minutes on each side or until golden brown and just cooked through.
10. Alternatively, grill over a hot grill after seasoning for 5-10 minutes on each side, again until easy cook ed through.
11. Easily remove chicken and set aside to cool.
12. Drain kelp noodles after 40to 45 minutes soaking in the water.
13. Add to the vegetables and toss with your hands or salad tongs.

14. Easy cut chicken in bite-sized pieces and add to salad.
15. Add dressing and toss again.
16. Serve now or chill, covered overnight.

www.ingramcontent.com/pod-product-compliance
Lightning Source LLC
Chambersburg PA
CBHW060701030426
42337CB00017B/2705